PARENTING ADHD
WITH WISDOM & GRACE

A guide to parenting and building
a positive relationship with your
child one moment at a time

Tish Taylor, PhD

FORWARD PRESS
OVERLAND PARK, KS.

First published in 2019 by Forward Press.
Cover Design by Lesley Ehlers.
All right reserved by Tish Taylor, Ph.D.
www.tishtaylor.com

All rights reserved. No part of this publication may be reproduced, distributed, or transmitted in any form or by any means, including photocopying, recording or other electronic or mechanical methods, without the prior written permission of the publisher, except in the case of brief quotations embodied in reviews and certain other non-commercial uses permitted by copyright law.

ISBN-10: 0-9842725-0-X
ISBN-13: 978-0-9842725-0-1

*To my husband, children, and family:
I love you.*

*To Dr. Robert Harrington:
Thank you for believing in me.*

Contents

Chapter 1	I'm Overwhelmed!	1
Chapter 2	At this Rate, We're in Trouble	9
Chapter 3	Where Do I Start?	17
Chapter 4	Embarrassing Parenting Moments	31
Chapter 5	I've Lost My Confidence	43
Chapter 6	Will My Child Ever Learn?	55
Chapter 7	This Behavior is Unacceptable	65
Chapter 8	I Need Help	75
Chapter 9	I'm an Over-Functioning Parent	87
Chapter 10	My Child Is a Gift	99

CHAPTER 1

I'm Overwhelmed!

Sophie is a wife and mother of three children, one with ADHD. She comes home after work and quickly goes through her mental checklist of what needs to be done that evening. She needs to figure out something to fix for dinner (as she forgot to plan ahead), pick up one child from volleyball practice and another from music lessons within half an hour of each other, fix dinner and do the dishes after, follow up with a phone call from work, call her mother back, and make sure that all homework is completed and everyone's school materials and backpacks are ready for tomorrow. While Sophie isn't a stressed person by nature, her busy life and never-ending to-do list can make her that way on any given day.

When it comes time to check on homework, her son Alex, immediately begins to argue. He insists that he doesn't have any, so she doesn't need to check. Homework is a trigger word for Alex. It equates to immediate resistance and arguing. Sophie thinks to herself, "Are you kidding? I know that you at least have math homework and a spelling test on Friday. Do you talk to your teachers like this? What in the world are you going to say when you have a job? Are you going to talk to a boss like this? If so, you won't have a job for long!"

But she doesn't say any of this out loud. Instead, she stops, takes a breath, and thinks about what is most pertinent in this moment: getting Alex through this moment of resistance as peacefully as possible. She strives to do so without creating a power struggle or adding to an already long day. So, she says, "Alex, we review your homework every night. The same goes for your brother and sister. This is routine for all of us." She goes on, lightheartedly, "Let's check anyway just to be sure." As Alex continues to protest, she coaxes gently and moves forward with checking the online system for homework, letting him know through her actions that this is an expected routine.

Sophie has learned that when she stays focused on one specific action at a time and keeps Alex focused on one specific step at a time, they both get through the situation with less conflict and decrease the likelihood of an outburst. While it takes all of her patience in that moment, Sophie knows that dealing with an outburst would take far more energy. When she avoids an outburst and Alex is better able to cope, she feels some hope for him and their situation.

In the above scenario, Sophie remembered the adage *this is one moment in time.* Remembering this adage can bring levity to any stress-filled situation. Whatever "it" is that is happening, it will not last forever. At some point in the future—maybe in the very near future—the circumstances may feel quite different. Reminding ourselves that it is only one moment in time helps us to avoid responding in an overly emotional way.

As a parent, it is normal to think about your child's future. Our minds naturally wander, thinking, "I hope he will be able to manage" or "I hope she doesn't have to learn the hard way" or "He better learn this now." I believe that this foresight is important, because we need perspective about our child's traits and what they can eventually mean for his or her future. However, it is equally important to keep these projections balanced. When we focus too much on shortcomings or weaknesses, we introduce stress into our parenting. For example, when anxiety becomes a part of our projections, we tend to overly focus on the negative. This can create more pressure and bring overwrought emotion into parenting and parent–child interactions.

In all honesty, you know that your child with ADHD has specific difficulties for which there is no cure. You go through times when your child is not organized, forgets the easiest things with predictable consequences, or doesn't respond to or seem to learn from repeated consequences. Again, remembering that these situations are all *one moment in time* can lighten the frustration and stress. Your child's entire future does not hinge on this one moment. And you are unlikely to change your child's entire future in this one moment. But you can continue to guide, teach, and build upon a positive relationship with your child in one moment. Over time, these interactions work toward improving ADHD traits and can help you parent through some difficult situations.

You may be saying, "You should be living my life." You may feel that maintaining a peaceful inner self and dealing with frustrating situations every single day is more than you are humanly able to do. And this is understandable. However, try to imagine taking a breath and remembering that the world is not going to come shattering down in this one circumstance. Could you then live through this moment for what it is? *One moment in time.* Who knows? Maybe this moment could be one of your best parenting moments. There may be benefit not only to your child but also to you.

Another point to remember is that a relationship built upon love, respect, and dignity will serve your child for the rest of his or her life. In so many ways, a parent–child relationship that has many positive facets will benefit a child now and in the future. I am not suggesting that you refrain from providing guidance, correction, or even consequences when needed. What I am suggesting is that you do so with emotional self-control and clarity.

Present or Future?

Present thinking is defined as thinking that is in the present moment. It includes those salient features of the circumstance without adding more to the situation than is warranted. *Future thinking* is defined as thinking that projects ahead in time. In this context, I am referring to future thinking as projecting ahead in time regarding your child's future.

For example, when your child plays in the neighborhood, you may notice that his or her impulsive behavior annoys other children. You begin to worry about these friendships and think "the friend group will be smaller next year" or "I hope these kids will still want to play with him in the future." Another example of future thinking would be concern about negative repercussions if your child's GPA is below a 3.0. This may sound like "she won't attend her dream school if she doesn't step it up."

Are these future thoughts aligned with likely future outcomes? Well, probably. But can we totally predict the future? *No.* So, trying to remain mindful and recognizing when you slip into future thinking may help you return to a focus in the present. Present thinking allows us to address the behavior or specific circumstance in the moment as opposed to resorting to a lecture or an overwrought response.

For example, you might be tempted to say, "You really should think about your behavior because other kids will not want to hang around you if you keep acting like that." Then, when your child scoffs at this, you respond, "Hey, I'm just trying to help you." But does that really help? Instead, consider saying something focused specifically on the present situation, such as, "Did you notice how Marcus rode his bike away from you when you popped a wheelie right next to him? Did you see how that made him uncomfortable?" This type of comment provides greater clarity and social awareness for the situation in the moment, as opposed to predicting a negative future outcome from a behavior that your child may not have recognized.

Future thinking is also reflected in comments like, "You really need to think about your GPA and how it will affect attending your dream school" or "You better get this done if you want to meet your goals." Instead, you may have a better outcome by considering the present moment and saying "I can see that you are overwhelmed. I'll help you make a plan for tonight's homework so that you can get it finished in time to talk to your friends."

Can you totally escape future thinking? No. Should you totally avoid future thinking about your child? No. However, if future thinking is increasing your reactivity, escalating the intensity beyond what the situation warrants, and leading to unhelpful responses, a shift to present thinking can help. Taking a breath and considering one moment in time can allow for a more measured and wiser response to the situation, ultimately guiding your child or teen toward a more positive future outcome.

Chapter Tips

- One moment or situation will not make or break your child's entire future.
- Addressing a specific behavior can be more helpful than communicating worry about the future.

- Maintaining a connection with your child is more likely when you understand them in any given moment.
- You are in this for the long haul, one moment at a time.
- Do you best with the moment you have in any given circumstance.

CHAPTER 2

At this Rate, We're in Trouble

Parenting your child is a journey. It is accomplished day by day, week by week, month by month, and year by year. During this process, growth patterns can sometimes seem to stall, while at other times, seem to jump ahead quickly. This is not atypical. So, don't worry if something is not improving or developing immediately. However, if an important skill or trait doesn't seem to *ever* improve, then it's time to review your approach, change your plan, and find the right help. Remember, *it's a journey*.

Consider the analogy of growing and tending to a lawn. There is the initial major effort in seeding the lawn and getting the grass to grow, which must be followed by ongoing maintenance. And no matter the stage of the lawn's growth, conditions are usually less than perfect and may even be extreme (such as not enough or too much rain, too hot or too cold, weeds taking hold). Tending the lawn under these changing conditions takes time and effort, more so when conditions are not the same for the entire lawn, which is likely. Additional tending will be needed for some areas, such as a low-lying area that becomes overwatered or an unshaded area burning out in the summer sun. Similar to tending to an entire lawn, tending to the entire development of a child requires continual vigilance, nurturing, and accommodating different circumstances and characteristics. At times, your child may be moving forward in a positive direction (just like grass shooting up in the spring), while at other times, not as much. However, within this journey, you should continually strive to move forward as much as you can while working with the many variables and changing conditions.

As you gain more experience with your lawn, you'll become better at anticipating and tending to the particular challenges that arise. Again, in parenting, it is similar. There is a continual nurturing, anticipating what may be coming, and managing circumstances when they come up. But you should always keep in mind that any particular challenge is temporary. A patch of lawn that is water-soaked won't remain that way forever, and neither will a difficult situation with your child. More than that, by cultivating the more successful practices as you go, you'll learn what nurtures your child most effectively.

I urge you to stay true to your overarching goals for your child, even during frustrating or exacerbating circumstances. Do not ignore what needs to be addressed, but when your child has a bad day, or other tough time or setback, remember to stay on the path of parenting for positive outcomes. Do not become overwhelmed by thoughts of negative or *"what if"* outcomes. 'What if your child never grows out of this behavior? What if he or she stays like this for the foreseeable future?" Again, remember this is a journey and do your best to maintain a balanced perspective.

The Big Picture

What is the big picture? I think of it as a snapshot, or a map, of a child's entire growth and development from infancy to adulthood. On this big picture map, some sections are smoother than others, some sections have large and treacherous hills (harder times), and some sections include a little downhill trail (easier times). As in life, situations and circumstances ebb and flow. However, do not forget that it is all part of the journey that you take as a parent and a family. Keeping this visual in mind is a good way to allow you to see that any one moment is a very small part of the entire journey. Some larger events may alter the course on the map, but nothing is fully written or determined until it actually happens.

Think about the "end of the journey" or some point when your child is on his own in adulthood. What do you envision? That he will be happy and healthy? That he will be engaged in an occupation or work activity that is fulfilling and uses his abilities? Or maybe you just envision gainful employment so that your child can live independently (and not in your basement). Whatever this vision is for you, hold on to it. If you have not taken some time to envision this, do so now. Being connected to an end goal is important to help you maintain focus over the years. Realize where you are headed and that each day or situation can help guide you there. Although sometimes it may not seem like you are making progress, by using your insight and what you learn about what is effective and what is not, you will eventually reach the end you have envisioned.

An important point about your envisioned end goal is that it will need to be fluid. If you make the goal too specific (eg, my child will go to college, graduate and then attend graduate school), you are writing your child's future for him or her. A better vision is one that is targeted but yet still open to different possibilities. For example, "My child will be an independent and functioning adult" or "My child will find work that she enjoys."

Your understanding of your child's strengths and abilities will certainly influence the shape and focus of the overall vision. However, as children age, especially into their teen years, they will want to have more and more input about their future goals. This is another reason for keeping end goals open to different opportunities.

Values

The specific larger goals and desires you identify for your child should align with your overall values. When you truly think about it, goals are embedded within values. Often, values are related to treatment of self and others, personal responsibility and accomplishments, relationships and family, faith and spirituality, citizenship or civic responsibility, individual pursuits and fulfillment, etc. When considering overall goals for your child, you may also think about the values these goals exemplify and why you believe them to be important.

Notice the values rooted within these examples of larger goals:

- Alex will develop his strengths and talents to the best of his ability.

- Alex will gain insight and understanding about how to help himself stay organized.
- Alex will learn to respect himself and others.
- Alex will take responsibility for himself and his actions.
- Alex will successfully complete his high school or college education.
- Alex will be gainfully employed as an adult.
- Alex will function proficiently within his relationships.

Scenario

Alex is not organized. He has never been organized. His parents describe him as going through the apartment like a Tasmanian devil. He forgets worksheets from school, misplaces his shoes for soccer practice, and often loses his key to the apartment. His parents have spent countless hours trying to find the "right" planner, binder, and other organizational materials to help him. He either doesn't keep up with them or loses them. It may start out well for a week or so, but progress is quickly lost. Before you know it, he is missing some assignments and his parents are scrambling to find out what is now due or past due.

His parents say, "We have tried everything. We have tried every planner on the market. We have sat with him. We have reminded him constantly. Why isn't he making progress? Is he ever going to get it?"

Alex has an obvious organizational deficit related to ADHD. A combination of efforts will likely be needed to allow him to function as best as he can organizationally. Remember, this is a journey. Part of the journey for Alex and his parents is finding what combination of interventions and accommodations will work best for Alex—and ultimately for Alex to eventually use those interventions for himself.

Chart Your Course

Alex and his parents certainly experience struggles on a daily basis. However, maintaining a perspective that allows for learning, including trial and error learning, while staying focused on overarching goals and values will provide more fruitful outcomes. The saying "Rome was not built in a day" has stood the test of time because it embraces wisdom and truth. Major changes or development always occur over time. We often become flummoxed when we see behaviors that need to change but do not. In reality, when dealing with a neurodevelopmental disorder, change will not occur overnight. Some areas may not fully change, but they can improve. Chart your course by staying focused on the big picture. The small positive steps you make in the short term will add up and keep you on the path to your envisioned outcome.

Chapter Tips

- See the bigger picture while living the present.
- Be secure and clear about your parenting values.
- Identify goals that are aligned with your values.
- Allow yourself to be flexible with your goals as you continue to understand your child.
- Embrace the positive growth and changes at the same time you are experiencing the frustrations and challenges.

CHAPTER 3

Where Do I Start?

As a busy parent, I often find myself thinking "what do I still need to finish so that I can get through this day?" or often more simply "is it Friday yet?" Many of our thoughts are short term, focused on what is right in front of us. However, while you're juggling all your to-do items, it may be helpful to consider your vision and overall goals for your child as part of the present. *Embedding longer term goals into the present is different than future thinking discussed in the previous chapter.* What we are talking about here is based on specific goals and outcomes that are both targeted and directed. It is not rooted in worry, emotions, and negative outcomes. Rather, it is driven by values. If you keep your greater vision and long-term goals in mind, you can think about in-the-moment behaviors that will lead toward the desired direction. This focus will help you to teach and guide appropriately as situations arise.

Scenario

> Jaden is a bright student. He is meeting all the curricular objectives for his grade, and his teachers have not had any major concerns. However, Jaden's mom, Melanie, is concerned because it's becoming difficult to get Jaden to do homework or any type of academic task outside the school day. She notices that he dislikes reading and that, when he does read, he has trouble focusing on reading more than a paragraph and doesn't seem to be paying attention. Jaden claims that he cannot remember anything that he reads. However, he seems to remember many, many other things, and there are no obvious signs of memory difficulties. He puts up a fight and finds various ways to procrastinate doing any type of reading, including the 20-minute nightly reading expected by his teacher.
>
> Melanie knows that Jaden has the ability to remain a strong student and envisions him completing high school and attending college. However, resisting and avoiding reading is not a step in that direction. So, she is thinking about some short-term goals that may support

the longer-term educational goal. Finding ways to motivate Jaden to read may include identifying books that he finds more interesting, asking his teacher to encourage nightly reading, using a reward system for reading, making reading a special time that she and Jaden share together, making reading time the same time each day so that it becomes expected in their routine, and allowing for screen time only after reading is completed.

Melanie stays focused on long-term goals and short-term strategies because she values Jaden's learning and future education. She finds that continuing to motivate Jaden to read is needed to keep his academic skills at a level that will allow him to be successful in the future.

What Do You Value?

Think about what is most important to you and the values you want to instill in your child. These values should drive your parenting. What do you want to accomplish as a parent? What do you want your child to value as an adult? Considering your most important values is very helpful to guide your parenting. Below is a list of some common values:

- Respect for self
- Respect for others
- Compassion
- Independence
- Persistence
- Reliability
- Faith
- Responsibility
- Social responsibility
- Confidence
- Creativity
- Morality
- Competence
- Honesty

While this list is not exhaustive, it does provide a flavor of family and individual values. You may also consider the question, "as an adult, I want my child to clearly recognize what I believe to be important in life." Give this a great deal of thought.

Once you have determined a range of values, you can use them to derive your goals. Your goals should be closely aligned with your values, which are purposeful and enriching. Knowing your goals will help you communicate with your child in a way that is driven by values rather than by emotional reaction. Assuming that respect is an important value, consider how you might instill respect in your child if he or she has emotional outbursts or temper tantrums. Please do not misunderstand—emotions are part of life, being human, and of course, parenting. Emotions can inspire and convey feelings, but emotions can also overwhelm and not have good judgment or lead to the best decisions. Your parenting choices should be guided by your values and not by emotion.

Developing Short-Term Goals and Action Steps

Once you have clearly determined your most important values, consider how to translate them into goals and action steps. This will guide your ability to respond in various situations. To better illustrate this, here are a few examples of short-term goals and action steps for Alex (introduced in Chapter 2) that mirror larger goals and values.

- Alex will be gainfully employed as an adult. The long-term goal is based on values of independence, confidence, and reliability.
    - Alex will complete 2 or 3 household chores weekly.
    - Alex will complete his homework.
    - Alex will learn to communicate his thoughts and, at times, compromise.
    - Alex will develop self-confidence.

- Alex will develop his strengths and talents to the best of his ability. The long-term goal is based on values of competence, persistence, and responsibility.
    - Alex will engage in extracurricular activities that he enjoys.
    - Alex will follow through with the "rigor" (practice, responsibilities, etc) of extracurricular activities.
    - Alex will complete assigned school work with quality.
- Alex will gain insight and understanding about how to help himself. The long-term goal is based on values of independence, confidence, and competence.
    - Alex will learn organizational strategies.
    - Alex will communicate what tasks are more difficult for him.
    - Alex will be able to communicate and strategize when he knows something is more difficult for him.
    - Alex will recognize his high-energy level and use methods to help regulate it.
- Alex will learn to respect himself and others. The long-term goal is based on the value of respect.

- Alex will speak using respectful language.
- Alex will talk about himself in a dignified manner.
- Alex will show gratitude and consideration toward others.
* Alex will successfully complete his high school or college education. The long-term goal is based on values of independence, competence, and persistence.
    - Alex will pass his classes with at least average grades.
    - Alex will complete at least 95% of his assigned work (this can be a tall order for a child with ADHD!)
    - Alex will communicate with his teachers when he has a question or is having difficulty.
    - Alex will adhere to a homework routine.
    - Alex will adhere to using an organizational system.
* Alex will function proficiently within his relationships. The long-term goal is based on values of respect and compassion.
    - Alex will be able to enjoy time with others with minimal conflict.
    - Alex will show dignity for himself and others.

- - Alex will develop proficient interpersonal communication skills.
  - Alex will increase his awareness skills and consider others' perspectives.
- Alex will take responsibility for himself and his actions. The long-term goal is based on values of responsibility, reliability, and social responsibility.
  - Alex will accept responsibility for his own actions.
  - Alex will follow directions to complete his responsibilities.
  - Alex will consider his choices before acting on impulses.
  - Alex will recognize when he has hurt someone and apologize.
  - Alex will keep words and actions safe, even when he is upset.
  - Alex will use calming strategies and practice self-control in frustrating moments.

This list likely feels overwhelming. Do not let it. It is simply meant to provide some examples that may fit your situation or that you can use to create your own. Start by choosing one, two, or three relevant goals and/or action steps. It's true that even one aspect of a goal may take much of your parenting time, so it may help to consider what is most valued or needed right now. Doing so will help guide your thoughts, efforts, and awareness in a positive and goal-specific direction. You will be tuned into resources, strategies, or even a comment made by another person that could be helpful. Keeping your efforts proactive instead of reactive will bring value into teachable moments.

Focus on Growth

As you consider your specific goals, remaining focused on what you want to nurture, encourage or grow will lead you in a positive direction. For example, if your child is quick to interrupt conversations, then aim to develop a "pause button." Focus on what would help your child develop more awareness by checking social cues and indicating when to ask a question or enter into a conversation. Just thinking about the term "pause button," helps steer in the right direction of what you're trying to encourage.

To further this example, think holistically about how you could encourage, support and teach this behavior. Teaching this skill and encouraging it within specific interactions could include any or all of the following:

- Teaching a visual cue to stop, look, and take in the social cues
- Teaching a visual cue to wait a moment
- Modeling this behavior within your family
- Providing encouragement when your child tries to stop and check social cues
- Reminding your child about this social skill before company arrives
- Modeling and encouraging this behavior by teachers or other prominent individuals in your child's life

These are just a few of many examples. The point is to broaden your thinking about all the ways this skill could be developed or at least improved.

When considering how you can holistically address your valued goals, think about what would encourage and reinforce the desired skills. Is something missing that is hindering skill development? Are there concentrated efforts that would help improve the skill?

Let's go back to the example of Jaden and his reading homework. The strategies mentioned included increasing positive motivation, creating a mindset of expectation, setting up consistent practice, and even creating an emotional comfort surrounding reading practice. Jaden's mother thought about different aspects of his environment,

Where Do I Start?

as well as how to build more confidence and encouragement around Jaden's reading behaviors.

The figure below will help you envision and target specific skills by thinking about the factors that influence development of a skill or ability. Consider different aspects of the home environment, outside environment, family habits, your child's specific traits, and anything that may be hindering development of a particular skill. Parenting a child with ADHD often requires determining how to address each of these aspects systematically to progress in a positive direction.

Center: Targeted Skill

- How are home practices supporting the skill?
- How are outside influences supporting the skill?
- How are parenting practices supporting the skill?
- How are my child's behaviors and abilites supporting the skill?

Think about a recent or common situation and what specific strategies you could use and if there are other ways you could intercede. Practicing this in your mind helps before something actually happens because you will likely need to change your behavior or respond differently than you have in the past. Remember, both you and your child have a learning curve! Keep your directions, reminders, and even visual cues short and to the point. Try not to lecture your child, because this generally decreases progress toward a specific behavior. A better option is an effective cue or a one-sentence reminder. In addition, be sure that your nonverbal communication, including your facial expression, eye contact, tone, and body language, appear confident and non-threatening. This is a lot to think about, so practicing how it sounds and looks will be helpful. It is natural to fall back on your past parenting responses. Parenting in even a slightly different style will require persistent practice and, along with continued self-reflection, will lead to lasting parenting changes.

Are We There Yet?

To be honest, achieving 100% of the goal may not be realistic. But keep in mind the improvement you are striving for. For example, if the frequency or intensity of a certain behavior decreases, that is progress! You are closer to the goal than you would be if you hadn't made a concerted effort. And during the process of striving to improve a behavior, you'll learn what may be more or less effective in a given situation. The more knowledgeable you become in understanding your child and his or her behaviors and reactions, as well as your own, the closer you will both come to positive outcomes.

Chapter Tips

- Think about your parenting values and write them down.
- Think about short term goals for your child, which are grounded in your values, and write them down.
- Prioritize what goals are in most need of attention.
- Evaluate what factors are facilitating growth and impeding progress.
- Celebrate the successes.

CHAPTER 4

Embarrassing Parenting Moments

How many times do you get "the look" from others? A family member, a friend, or even a stranger! How many times do you receive unsolicited parenting advice? The theme is often around disciplining your child with ADHD. Others may observe your child talking back, being sassy or disrespectful, refusing to follow directions or procrastinating, or generally acting inappropriately. You may provide a reasonable explanation such as "he's extra tired today" or "this type of situation is hard for her." But, honestly, you need to deal with the behavior firsthand and sometimes you may feel like responding in a manner that would land child protective services at your door. In these instances, you may feel judgment, pity, or maybe even confusion from others. None of this does much for your parenting confidence and, in turn, makes it uncomfortable to be around those who offer advice and judgement.

Is there something else that you can say or do in these situations? Yes, there is! However, let's start with clearly understanding what is happening in these moments.

What Are We Talking About?

First and foremost, let's clarify common ADHD traits and simple ways to label them. It helps to understand what you are dealing with in uncomfortable parenting moments. The following is a list of some of the most common and problematic traits that accompany ADHD. It is not exhaustive and every child will not have every trait to a significant degree, but you will likely relate to many of them.

- *Sense of time*: lacking an ability to judge how much time is needed and how much time is left, and the sense or urgency to "hurry up"
- *Mental shift*: difficulty mentally accepting and shifting from one activity to another, especially to non-preferred activities
- *Emotional reactivity*: displaying a greater than expected or even extreme emotional reaction given the situation

- *Acceptance of authority*: recognizing that an adult direction needs to be accepted and followed without ignoring, negotiating, or arguing
- *Task initiation*: difficulty starting tasks in a timely manner
- *Task completion*: difficulty staying focused long enough or being organized enough to complete a task, or with completing a task on time
- *Difficulty accepting "no" or not getting one's way*: this tends to go on much longer than would be expected given a child's chronological age
- *Distractibility*: not starting or completing tasks because of internal or external distractions
- *Organization*: losing materials and important things, leaving a mess, and/or having difficulty managing school and home responsibilities

When you put all or at least some of these together, it is easy to see how they can converge into a disciplinary, parenting nightmare, especially if outside the home or around others. Don't forget that fatigue, lack of nutrition, stress, or a generally agitated mood will heighten the intensity of these situations.

Find Clarity within Yourself

First and foremost, it is important to clarify your intentions and goals. Communicating with others is difficult if you do not have internal clarity. Think back to your vision, values, and goals. How might you integrate them into any given situation? What are you trying to nurture? What is your goal in this situation? What is the most important aspect of this situation? Considering these questions will help you develop a clearer thought process and, in so doing, clearer communication.

Scenario

Sarah and her 12-year-old daughter, Erin, went to Target for a typical shopping trip, which they have affectionately termed the "Target Run." Erin had visions of buying a new accessory for her phone and, although she had briefly mentioned something about it earlier in the week, Sarah had had a lot on her mind and just wasn't thinking about it. When they entered the store, Erin quickly told her mother that she wanted to go to the electronics aisle to look at the phone accessories. Sarah agreed and said they'd meet in the grocery section. When Erin came back with the phone accessory, Sarah said "no, not today." Erin became angry immediately and started to argue. "Why? You let Luke have one. That's not fair!" Given Erin's volatile reaction and the fact that she was starting to make a scene in public, Sarah became frustrated. So, she grit her teeth and told Erin to put the accessory back where it belonged with a firm "no." With that, Erin stomped off without a word. Sarah finished her shopping and began searching through the aisles for Erin, who was nowhere to be found. At this point, Sarah began to worry because she had no idea where Erin was, or even if her daughter had remained in the store. She decided to pay for her items and return to her car to see if Erin was in the parking lot. Erin was indeed sitting on the curb by the car, but Sarah didn't feel much better as it was getting dark outside. She was ready to wring her daughter's neck...

In this scenario, Sarah had to think quickly, clearly identify, and communicate the most salient issues in the situation. How do you communicate clearly with your child—not just the issue but also the expected behavior in the moment? Parenting a pre-teen is already challenging and, in the above scenario, Sarah's daughter also exhibits emotional intensity and reactivity, as well as poor coping skills by having an outburst when told "no." She did not exhibit safe behavior by deciding to go to the car by herself. She didn't let Sarah know that she intended to leave the store, and so there wasn't time to communicate further about a possible purchase. Sarah could handle this situation by saying something like, "I'm upset because returning to the car in the dark without letting me know was not a safe choice. Plus, I didn't have time to think about your request. I felt 'put on the spot' and embarrassed because other people were noticing." These types of statements communicate safety, respect, and dignity. Consider as in this example how to target specific behaviors with values and goals—and how to do so without a lecture.

Sarah's daughter did not calm down right away. She still felt the situation was unfair because her brother had recently been allowed to get the same item. However, Sarah understands that her daughter will not likely see her perspective right away. She knows that her daughter needs more time to settle her emotions and to gain some insight into the situation and her behavior. Sarah can also tell her daughter that they will discuss the desired phone accessory after they talk about safe and respectful behaviors.

Scenario

Mary told her 13-year-old son, Steven, that it was time to come inside and finish his chores. Steven screamed "shut up, Mom!" in response, well within earshot of a couple of neighbors. Mary was mad. She felt that Steven's behavior was embarrassing and disrespectful and that it left a terrible impression with the neighbors. Mary wanted to prevent the situation from escalating any further. She clearly and calmly insisted that Steven was to come in the house now. Once he was inside, she instructed him to go to his room so that they both had some time to cool off. Even though it was extremely difficult to remain calm, Mary knew that a yelling fest would not help. She instructed Steven to stay in his room (without use of his phone, screens, etc) until he was ready to accept responsibility for his behavior and discuss the situation.

Mary's first words were, "are you ready to talk to me?" Steven responded, "I don't know." Because Mary can read Steven's moods and his ability to reason in the moment, she could tell that he was currently more receptive to a discussion than when he is in an intense emotional state. (If that had been the case, she would have waited a while longer.) She started by saying, "I felt hurt and disrespected because of what you said to me and how it was said." Her tone conveyed some disappointment but was firm and composed to avoid potentially spiking the situation again. Because Mary had waited until Steven was calm and thinking outside of his emotion, he begrudgingly apologized but followed quickly with a loud "But you interrupted my game! You do that all the time. This was my time, and you took it away from me." Mary replied, "We can address your feelings about this situation in a moment. However, first and foremost, the language and tone used with me was not respectful." Once Steven genuinely apologized, Mary then acknowledged his feelings and why he felt that way. She coached him to communicate differently in the future with the following: "You could have said: 'Mom, I'm frustrated because you said that I had free time and you didn't tell me that I had to do any chores.'" She reminded him that when he communicates respectfully, she will listen, but that he must also listen to her response for their communication to be effective.

In this situation, Mary believed that establishing respect was the priority. Steven's feelings and management of his feelings did not trump the level of disrespect he had shown. While he does need to understand and work through his feelings and figure out how to handle them differently, he needs to learn that respect and respectful language come first. Mary believes that this is of utmost importance and was firm with this value.

It is important to understand that this scenario played out the way it did because there is an established respect between Mary and Steven. Steven has emotional outbursts and gets angry in what seems like a split second, but Mary has nurtured a loving and respectful relationship with him over the years. She also maintains respect within their home, modeling respectful behavior with his siblings, others, and herself. If the home environment included disrespectful language, insults, yelling, and other forms of angry communication, this situation likely would not have ended this way.

If you identify a lack of respect in your home or within your relationships, then it is important to seek professional assistance.

I Feel Judged

What do you say to the judgmental in-law or eye rolling neighbor?

First, remain confident in your values and your parenting. No one parents perfectly all the time, and you know that you are doing your best.

You can always engage in active self-reflection about your parenting and ways to improve interactions with your child. However, you know and understand your child, your family circumstances, and what will work and not work in given situations better than anyone else. You do not have to be boorish when responding to the doubting onlooker but respond in a manner that maintains your dignity and that of your family.

Second, focus on how you need to parent your child in this situation. Do not allow others to unduly influence you if you are not comfortable with their suggestions or expectations. If the situation is uncomfortable and you are in someone else's home or space, then graciously find a way to allow the situation to settle.

If, however, you are struggling to feel confident in parenting your child, you may want to seek advice from a trusted family member or friend. It could also be a sign that you need more knowledge or professional assistance. Recognize that under the right circumstances, seeking extra advice or support shows strength, not weakness.

Parenting unwanted behaviors in front of others is stressful, uncomfortable, and embarrassing to you and your child. It is not easy. You may feel like you are a failing parent, or that you are failing in that instance. Because parenting is such a personal role, judgement from others can feel intense, uncomfortable, and offensive. Stay focused on what you want to accomplish. Stay focused on clear communication with your child. The way you handle the situation will communicate volumes to another person.

Situations may come up when you feel that you need to say something to others. Consider keeping it short and focused on only what you want to reveal. You may listen to advice, support, or even sympathy. But when it comes to how much you reveal, be clear about the level of shared information that you believe is appropriate for you, your child, and your family. You could lead (and possibly end) with "Today is one of those parenting days..." or "thank you for understanding and being supportive" or "He's still learning..."

Do it with Confidence

Again, doing this is not easy. You'll need to feel self-respect and confident in maintaining respect among other family members and all of your relationships. Remember that no one else fully understands the complete and intimate picture of raising a particular child other than the one who is doing it day to day. This doesn't mean that others at times can't offer some insight or a different perspective. So, work to not be offended by their words, advice, or maybe even judgment. Later on, in your own time, consider what was said and whether another perspective might have some merit. Beyond that, however, remain confident that as your child's parent, you have the most complete insight and can make the best decisions within the big picture.

Chapter Tips

- Recognize the underlying ADHD deficits at play in any given situation.
- Think about how to address these deficits given your child's abilities in those areas while striving for learning and growth.
- In an intense or angry situation, focus on your values and the most important issues.
- Keep your communication short and focused on the most essential value and issue.
- Proceed confidently as you know your child and your family better than anyone.

CHAPTER 5

I've Lost My Confidence

Parenting a child with ADHD can elicit a crisis in confidence. It can feel overwhelming, frustrating, and confusing. I do not need to tell you that you are doing more for your child with ADHD than other parents are doing for their child without ADHD. You are managing not only your own "to-do" list, but also that of your child's. This often includes managing every last detail, such as making sure all homework is completed, that the homework is actually in your child's backpack, and that your child turns the homework in to the correct place when he or she is supposed to do so. Even though you may have covered most of the details, if you didn't follow up with every single one, something could be lost or left unfinished. Did I mention exhausting?

Many parents feel more irritable and less proactive than they would like to be. These feelings can translate into harried behavior and greater difficulty with your own mental and emotional health. It may not be possible to totally escape the sense of being overwhelmed, as it will happen periodically. The bigger issue is how to deal with your feelings so that you do not become less effective or feel less confident. How can you deal with this so that you do not become overbearing or end up constantly nagging?

Losing your confidence or feeling overwhelmed as a parent often makes you question yourself and leads to less decisiveness. In turn, this can blur your clarity when you make parenting decisions, which may then become more inconsistent. Inconsistent decisions translate to mixed messages and blurred boundaries for children, and the chance of unwanted behaviors increases.

Organize and Prioritize

One way to manage feeling overwhelmed is to practice keeping situations in perspective. First, consider what is the most important or what needs to be completed quickly or today. Is this the highest priority or at least high on the priority list? Is it something that has to be done now? Do you have to do it at all? It is perfectly reasonable to strive for what is most important or valued and not for perfection.

Second, find an effective organizational system that you like and use it regularly. Keeping track of family schedules and detailed "to-do" lists is a demanding task. Using daily, weekly, and monthly calendars can help you see what is going on now and in the near future. Calendars, planners, and reminder systems can keep you organized and prompted about what is coming up while you are managing what is happening right now. By keeping your calendars current and reviewing them frequently, you'll know how much time needs to be allotted for various tasks, and you can keep on top of things.

Third, think about what you can delete from your overall schedule or list. Is all of it truly necessary? Are all the "to-dos" leading yourself, your child, and your family in a valued direction? This type of reflection and assessment is important when managing the overall functioning of life and family. It may be difficult to cut something out, but maybe doing so will make a positive difference. Today's schedules are often so loaded with extracurricular activities and commitments that the sense of balance can be lost, tipping instead to frenzied and stressed. Consider whether you are maintaining a balance within the overall schedule for the well-being of everyone in your family. It is also worth remembering that parenting a child with ADHD takes more time—time that also needs to be factored into your day-to-day routine.

Scenario

Corinne works part-time and manages many of the household responsibilities, plus most of her three children's activities, which include sports, music lessons, school clubs, and drama practice. She finds ways to carpool, but nine different activities each week have her running around like an Uber driver. In addition to her marriage, her job, the household errands, school, and all the extracurricular activities, Corinne also has to keep up with her youngest son's day-to-day self-management because he has few to no organizational skills. He routinely forgets his homework materials, the necessary form for an upcoming field trip, or his shoes for soccer practice—and he isn't particularly bothered by any of it, including late assignments. This causes even more work, follow-up, and stress for Corinne.

It dawns on her one day that she needs to prioritize her family's activities and schedule. She thinks through what is most important for the family and for each child individually. What is really necessary for everyone's overall growth and well-being? What is not getting enough time? What is getting more time than it should? She decides to set up a daily organizational and management system for the family and for her youngest son and then to plan the day and week and pay specific attention to reviewing the calendar and to-do lists. Her new management plan also includes consistent communication with her son's teacher and school. Corinne is tired of constantly playing catch up and wants to have a more proactive system in place. Planning time for this type of system is a priority and will likely take less of her time once it is up and running. She also determines that her son needs to participate so that eventually, he will become more self-aware and responsible for managing himself.

Corinne doesn't want to take away activities or "short" her other children. So, she decides that for the time being, she'll have her youngest and middle child participate in the self-management and organizational check-in system both before and after school, but that it won't be necessary for her oldest child who is already quite independent and capable. After a month, Corinne will evaluate how this system is working and then make any needed adjustments.

In this scenario, Corinne pinpointed what was most problematic and came up with a reasonable intervention step that addressed a primary problem. She also determined an evaluation target date to decide if she will need to change anything about her system. Because she took the time to review her family's situation, made a decision about what she could do about it, and followed through with a plan, Corinne's confidence increased immediately.

Self-Care

The experience of a busy parent typically results in feeling tired and overwhelmed. Where was the energy you once had? How can you help yourself find more energy and more positive energy? Although we all know that we need to take care of ourselves and even "put on our oxygen masks before that of our child's," we often don't follow through with consistent practices of self-care.

The foundation of self-care has three components: a good diet, physical exercise, and a balanced sleep schedule. All three are essential for managing our physical energy level and our emotional and mental health. Think about how you can find space in your day to improve at least one of these areas. Is there anything you can do to specifically improve your diet or get more exercise or sleep? Maybe it is taking some time each week for meal planning or putting specific items on your grocery list. Maybe it is parking farther away when you stop at the school or the store, or contacting your neighbor for an early morning walk on the weekend. Maybe it is putting down your phone or skipping social media and getting ready for bed instead. Whatever it is for you, think seriously about at least one thing you can do to improve your self-care and then commit to it. The more you provide a healthy balance for yourself, the more room you create for positive energy and confidence.

Keep in mind that your self-care impacts not only you, but also your family. If you are not at your best or are gradually finding less positive energy to do what you need to do, that pattern can drag down everyone. On the other hand, if you have a positive balance in your physical and mental health, everyone will benefit. And, improvements in your self-care may spark the entire family's motivation for healthy habits.

Finally, remember that while diet, physical exercise, and sleep are critically important for everyone's brain health, they are especially so for an individual with ADHD. A key difficulty in ADHD is regulation, and by maintaining healthy habits yourself, you are modeling such behavior for your child with ADHD (and other family members). Thus, you are potentially increasing your effectiveness in managing ADHD.

Mental Management

Many terrific tools are available to help you manage emotions and decrease feelings of stress. Prayer and meditation practices are steeped in the human tradition and provide a sense of peace, inner strength, and wisdom. You also do them within your own mind, so no special equipment or location is needed. Because prayer and meditation allow a shift from the prefrontal cortex area of our brain, the area that focuses on goal-directed behavior, they help us reconnect with something greater and/or to a source of peace. This can be very helpful in setting a calmer, more positive mood and mindset, especially when we feel frustrated or overwhelmed.

Another option is to practice what is called mindfulness. Mindfulness is a popular secular practice that allows us to feel a deep sense of calm and to refocus on the body in the present moment. When we can shift out of our head and into our body, we can feel calm and allow our mind and body to rejuvenate. Once you learn to practice mindfulness, you can use these skills and techniques at almost any time or in any situation.

Some of my favorite resources for mindfulness and meditation include the following:

I've Lost My Confidence

- www.headspace.com/headspace-meditation-app (Headspace app)
- www.calm.com/ (Calm app)
- www.uclahealth.org/marc/mindful-meditations (guided meditations – UCLA)
- Various materials by Wayne Dyer
- Various materials by Jon Kabat-Zinn

Another important area of mental management includes our day-to-day and moment-to-moment thinking practices. Be aware and mindful of how you interpret different situations and what judgments you place on others or specific situations. Often, we think we don't know what to do, that we are out of ideas, or that we don't even know where to start with a problem. This type of thought process decreases our confidence. If you find yourself thinking these types of thoughts, remove them from your mind just like you would delete a file from your computer. You may not have a flash of brilliance right now, but more clues or answers will come up. Be open to what you may not have thought of yet. One technique, for example, is to consider what you would tell a close friend or maybe a sister who was feeling negatively about herself or her capabilities. Would you say, "You really don't have a clue, do you?" Of course you wouldn't (unless maybe as a joke). My rule is that if you wouldn't say it to someone you care about, then you shouldn't say it to yourself. So, now think about what you would say to a close friend who was feeling overwhelmed, stuck, or inept. Maybe you'd comment with something more along the lines of "I bet once you sleep on it, you'll be able to think of a couple of different options." Let that sink in and then say it to yourself. You will probably come up with something helpful or at least supportive to say. If you need to call a close friend to have him or her remind you how to talk to yourself in that way, then do so. But, ultimately, it is important to learn to do this for yourself.

Scenario

At the end of many days, Jasmin feels that while she managed to get herself and her children through the day ok, she didn't do so with the grace, style, and wisdom that she envisions. She secretly admits to herself that she nags a little more than she would like and that her "mom persona" is less than fun. Sometimes she worries that her children will be happy to leave when they are old enough. Is she doing something wrong? Is there something that she can do better? Can she be a more positive influence and source of energy with her children and family?

Being a source of positive energy only comes from finding it within yourself first. I love the quoted wisdom "you cannot give away what you do not have." It is crucially important to recognize that self-care, both physical and mental, is necessary for us to be our best. Positive mental well-being can spark more creativity, patience, and insight. Whatever you want to instill in your children in terms of character and positive traits, the most successful teacher is you.

Confidence, positivity, and self-care are all related. Choose one area in which you can make a specific improvement, put it into practice right now, and begin to feel the benefits.

Chapter Tips

- Evaluate your overall schedule and eliminate that which is not needed or valued.
- Create or maintain an organizational system for yourself and your family.
- Improve at least one area of self-care in regard to your diet, exercise, or sleep habits.
- Prioritize mental stress management through prayer and/or meditation.
- Practice kind and supportive self talk.

CHAPTER 6

Will My Child Ever Learn?

Scenario

Nolan has done it again! We have been through this scenario a million times, and he continues to forget. He just walked off and left his bookbag at the house again. Now, his homework and form that needed to be turned in today will be late or not accepted. I want to throw up my hands. I cannot be his laundress, secretary, tutor, and housekeeper for the rest of his life. He is going to have to take responsibility for himself. He will just have to suffer the consequences. His teacher says, just let him fail, he will learn. Maybe then he will learn. However, he doesn't seem to...

Scenario

I am at my wits end and have lost it with Samuel again! I just cannot handle his arguing and push back every time I give a direction. Not to mention a very basic direction that all other parents expect of their children. Today, he blew up at me for telling him it was time to turn off the Xbox. Why are basic directions so hard for him to handle? We go through this same thing all the time!

Breathe and Stay Focused on Your Goals

Breathe. Just breathe. "Put on your oxygen mask first." You are not alone in parenting these situations. These types of situations are what the journey of parenting ADHD entails. These behaviors do not fade away or self-correct the way they do with most other children. Remember that knee-jerk reactions are steeped in emotion and typically not productive.

The most common emotion felt in the scenarios above is frustration that is exacerbating. An angry, emotional response will add more conflict to an already charged situation that you will have to work to recover from later. So, stop and breathe. Take note of the situation and your escalated feelings, and then proceed more calmly and wisely. Remind your child of the skill you are trying to teach, such as reviewing his or her morning checklist, following through with steps to make up what he or she has forgotten, remembering the anger management skills worked on in therapy, or modeling and coaching how to respond when frustrated or disappointed.

You can be honest, clear, and direct in these situations, but it is important not to be condescending or shaming. Your job is to help your child through these moments and strive toward improvement while maintaining everyone's dignity and self-respect. If you are having a difficult time managing your own frustration, the fewer words the better. Return to your overall values and short-term goals. If a certain behavior happens time and time again, you know that is an area of focus for you and your child. If you have not considered how this repeated behavior fits into your overall value system and how to formulate a short-term goal, then do so now. It is much easier to handle moments like these when you have a clear mind about what you are striving to accomplish rather than venting your frustration.

In Nolan's scenario above, values of independence and competence are likely. This means that you value your child being able to do things for himself and become self-sufficient in developmentally appropriate ways. In regard to short-term goals, you may consider working toward an organizational system that improves the ability to remember and keep track of important items. Be sure to factor in the time to do so. You may also want to work toward a checklist system that becomes more automatic so that your child learns to rely on a helpful organizational strategy. If your child is old enough, you could also set a daily alarm reminder on his or her phone.

In Samuel's scenario above, we see values of respect and dignity in play. In this example, consider respect as not only Samuel respecting his parent, but also respecting himself and the family. One family member's blow up tends to bring down the entire family unit if other family members are nearby and become a part of the scene and mood. Remember also that actions towards one's self are part of what one *gives away* to others. If you *give away* disrespect, you are not demonstrating dignity for the other person, the situation, or for yourself. Samuel is also having difficulty accepting a direction, shifting from a preferred activity, and having difficulty with emotional regulation. He reacts much more than what would be expected given the circumstance and then has difficulty accepting that he did so, blaming it on others, and not understanding why others are upset with him.

Learning to stop and take a breath before responding would be a terrific goal. Learning to recognize disappointment in addition to frustration and anger would be another goal. Third, agreeing to calmly transition off the Xbox when time is up before beginning play could be another goal. This would provide a prompt for Samuel for appropriate behavior. There are varied examples of short-term goals, but the point is to think through and practice using more appropriate coping skills.

Notice Positive Change

When working toward behavior change, you are asking your child to find ways to reorganize their neural pathways. This will require small steps and *practice*. Be sure to recognize moments when your child seems to be trying or is at least moving in a positive direction. It's also important to recognize that your child may do better one day than on another. When learning something new that is not natural, progress is usually inconsistent. That is why it is important to stay focused on your goals and continue to model, reinforce positively, and recognize progress.

Reflection and Evaluation

If positive progress is very slow or lacking, take the time to clear your mind and think about what is happening. Do you need to modify your responses? Do you need to model the wanted or desired behavior more effectively? Are other people or circumstances reinforcing the negative behavior? Perhaps siblings keep agitating the situation or another adult is not on board with modeling the appropriate behavior? In this situation, typically some environmental factors are getting in the way of progress.

As another possibility, some internal factors may be interfering. Your child may not be motivated or see the need for change. He may perceive that he would be fine if you would just leave him alone. In these types of cases, accepting responsibility for self and behavior is an important goal. You may also consider professional help (if not already being sought) to address mindset and perspective taking. This could be in the form of individual or family therapy.

I urge you to not give up or feel hopeless. When people begin to feel this way, their efforts begin to lessen and any positive progress made is quickly lost. The situation may feel difficult, overwhelming, and impossible, but it is not. Yes, it is very hard, but it is not impossible.

I also urge you to modify your plan. Take some time to reflect on and evaluate your efforts and interventions, what their impact has been, and what has and has not been helpful. Consider what you could change and why. Then make the change and reevaluate.

The diagram below shows how you might think about this process. First, clearly define the trait or behavior that you are seeing, how it shows up, and what it looks like. Know it when you see it and interpret it for what it is. For example, it could be difficulty with any of the following: transitions, shifting stuck thinking, regulating feelings when disappointed or stressed, organizing and/or remembering day to day tasks, or following through and finishing a task. Second, consider your specific response. Third, what was the change or response to your action? Factor in any other specifics to the situation such as outside forces or others reacting at the same time and try to observe the result of your parental response to the behavior.

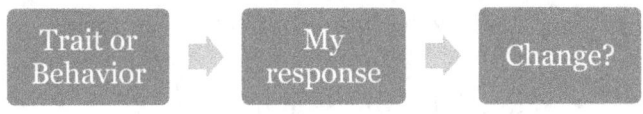

Sharpen Your Skills

ADHD traits and behavior patterns require more and varied parenting skills. Bottom line: applying all of the "standard" parenting skills or inclinations, including those that were modeled for you by your parents, are often not fully effective. I recommend using different resources to assist with increasing your understanding of ADHD traits and finding resources that increase your parenting skills when considering your particular child.

Important: ADHD traits do not present the same way in every child with ADHD. Each child with ADHD has a truly individual profile. It is also worth mentioning that there are severity levels to these traits. In some children, ADHD traits show up intermittently, while in other children, frequency and intensity of the ADHD traits are severe. Considering your child's specific profile will help you focus your efforts on what skills in your toolbox you need to improve or add.

The following materials provide excellent expert advice and techniques to help you develop ideas and strategies for challenging moments, as well as learn how to avoid ineffective scenarios:

- Materials by Russell Barkley
- Materials by Alan Kazdin
- Materials by Ross Greene
- *123 Magic* by Thomas Phelan
- *Parenting ADHD Now* by Elaine Taylor-Klaus and Diane Dempster
- *Smart but Scattered* materials by Peg Dawson and Richard Guare

Professional advice through individual or family therapy or parenting training classes is also helpful. Most psychologists and behavioral specialists working with children have training in ADHD and behavior management. Some social workers and counselors also have specific training and expertise in ADHD. However, before starting any therapy or classes, it is recommended to ask about the training and level of experience of the professionals in working with ADHD.

Chapter Tips

- ADHD is a diagnosis that indicates a slow learning curve in the deficit areas.
- You will find yourself trying to teach the same skill over and over, so focus on a positive goal.
- Notice your child's positive movement and effort.
- Closely observe and evaluate how your behavior impacts your child's behavior.
- Closely observe and evaluate how environmental factors or forces impact your child's behavior and adjust accordingly.

CHAPTER 7

This Behavior is Unacceptable

Scenario

Laken is bright and very capable of managing her schoolwork and a number of different activities. She has potential in many areas, but she can become inflexible and challenge authority, refuse to follow directions, and talk back to adults. If angered enough, she will walk off, throw something (possibly at someone), and insult or yell at whomever she perceived has wronged her. She does so without regard for any consequences and, at the time, believes her reactions are absolutely justified. She exhibits this behavior most often at home with her parents, but it has also occurred at school, sports practices, and social events like birthday parties. It is causing some major problems with both peers and adults. Laken has been placed on a behavior plan at school, and adult volunteers for activities have started avoiding having her on their teams. Sometimes, after Laken has had a chance to calm down, she feels remorse and does not like the consequences of her behavior. But she realizes this too late or, in some cases, still has difficulty understanding why others are upset with her.

Maintaining Dignity

This type of behavior has many challenging components. First, it sparks strong emotions among those involved. Adults anger quickly because of the disrespect, the aggression, and the outright refusal to follow directions. Their natural reaction to address a child showing this type of behavior is often strong, especially if someone could be harmed (physically or emotionally). When faced with this situation, most adults respond in an authoritative manner and try to take control of the situation. Laken's parents are not sure what to do because such strong responses intensify Laken's behavior and emotions, and the result is a huge power struggle. Everyone feels horrible both during and afterward.

This Behavior is Unacceptable

If this is your situation, you know how quickly it can erupt and catch you off guard. Think through how you will handle something like this before it happens again. Run through it your mind, say it out loud, and talk it over with your spouse, co-parent, or a trusted individual. By "practicing" ahead of time, you'll be able to respond more thoughtfully and carefully, which is not easy to do, especially when emotions are running high.

When these situations flare up, it's important to maintain as much dignity as possible for each person involved and for your family and others. The more dignity you can maintain, typically there is less regret and less "repair" work needed afterward. So, how do you do that? First, watch the words you use. Be sure to use language that *addresses the behavior and not the individual*. How something is expressed in words carries tremendous power in human interactions. The context and meaning of what is stated carry a great deal of impact, especially when emotions are high. Words that are harsh, unkind or hurtful require healing or repair work later. The more often such words are spoken, the deeper the scar or damage to the relationship.

Note the examples below and think about how the words used affect the level of dignity. Using words that target the behavior or skill help to maintain dignity, while those that are more personal and spoken in the course of frustration and anger do not. The latter results in a greater likelihood of negative feelings, both in the moment and that can linger long afterward.

More Dignity	**Less Dignity**
"Think about how others probably feel about it."	"You are not going to have any friends."
"Please, I need a minute as I am very upset."	"Shut up and leave me alone."
"That is argumentative, and it is not helping."	"Stop being such a jerk."
"Let's stop and take a breath."	"Shut your mouth."

Just as important as the words you use is what you convey through nonverbal communication—things like your tone of voice and body language. Even if you use more dignified words but say them with a tone of disgust or intense anger, you will communicate a negative message and feeling between yourself and your child. Both children and adults can sense the feeling behind nonverbal communication and tend to react quickly. If a parent's body language, through position, posture, or even a gesture, appears as if threatening to be physically forceful, the child's reaction is usually one of fight, flight or freeze. When a child is already in fight mode, it is easy to predict the outcome.

Remember to consider what your goal is in these situations. Maybe there is a need to establish control—and maybe for good reasons such as physical or emotional safety. But remember to do so while maintaining as much dignity as possible. Again, preserving dignity will mean less regret and repair work later after everyone has calmed down, allowing the greater focus to be on molding and shaping behaviors that need improvement. Although such improvement may be slow, in the end, you will have maintained a healthier relationship that will benefit both you and your child in the long run.

Shaming and Self-Esteem

Shaming essentially means using words and actions to communicate why a person should feel ashamed of himself or herself. It implies that someone is *bad* in some way. The problem with shaming is that it affects both self-concept (what I think about myself) and self-esteem (how I feel about myself), which can lead to feelings of inadequacy. When people feel this way, they often try to overcompensate around others by acting or pretending to be better than they believe they actually are. This behavior does not win any popularity contests in social interactions.

Shaming can elicit a different reaction in other individuals, resulting in more defiance, anger, or disrespect. These people do not accept the idea that they are bad, but instead conclude that *you* are bad or wrong. Consequently, their negative reaction becomes even stronger, creating a more difficult situation while not improving behavior.

Again, remember to separate the person from the action or the behavior. We all need to evaluate our behavior at times and be honest about what we may have done and need to do differently in the future. However, thinking about ourselves when we feel ashamed or when we believe that someone else is trying to make us feel "less than" is not helpful for personal growth.

Depending on their personality, children may show a high versus low self-esteem in regard to how they are perceived by others or what they think has occurred. Some children continue to believe in their own perspective, holding onto it and thinking that it is those around them who are causing the problem. These children do not seem to suffer from much regret or remorse, and they don't feel bad about themselves. Other children are less confident and have a more fragile self-esteem. Once a given situation is over and these children have calmed down, they feel remorseful and that they are "bad" or that others see them as "bad."

If you see your child in the first example, then building perspective around having concern for others is an important goal. If you see your child in the second example, then separating the behavior from the child, eliminating shaming, and teaching emotional regulation strategies are important goals.

Recovery

What to do when you have a less than stellar day of parenting? What if you have a less than stellar year of parenting? Many parents find that they become frustrated with ADHD traits and succumb to yelling or threatening to get their child to comply or complete a task. This can, in the moment, be effective in helping reach a short-term goal. However, if this becomes the main parenting technique, then the overall parent-child relationship suffers. The longer a parent uses negative parenting techniques, the more work will be needed to repair the parent-child relationship later.

If your parental responses are consistently angry or threatening, your child will learn to comply only under those conditions. In other words, your child will wait for the threat or negative interaction before responding and will not learn how to manage his or her own behavior without it.

If this is your situation, it's time to get started on repair work. If you know you could have handled a situation better, recognize and accept it, and then work to make it better. Do not let what you consider to be a failure or poor parenting discourage you from improving your parenting or parenting as you would like to.

A mother once told me that she had a "colossal failure" one night as her child was misbehaving. In the heat of the moment, she kept taking away more screen time until the punishment was far more than the behavior warranted. How many times have we over punished? This type of situation can be repaired by focusing on the positive behaviors we want to see and offering an alternative to meet the desired outcome. This technique allows children to recover from their poor choices and allows parents to recover from over punishing. It also allows redirecting to something more hopeful and motivating. In this example, the mother allowed quicker recovery of screen time once her child demonstrated being able to follow directions. The mother provided a clear and attainable path for the child to earn back screen privileges.

There are endless examples of parenting that may leave both you and your child feeling that it could have gone better or that the negative aspects of everyone's behavior in certain moments were not productive. Do not be discouraged! This happens

This Behavior is Unacceptable

to everyone. Working to correct or improve a circumstance *can* be done. Take the time and maintain your focus on working toward the positive behaviors and traits that you are trying to cultivate in your child.

A final note: If you have more instances of parent-child interactions that have ended in major arguments, hurt feelings, and regret, then consider seeking outside therapy support to mend and build a stronger relationship between you and your child. You may also consider parenting classes to help you learn and practice different skills. You will likely need to learn new, more and different skills when parenting a child with ADHD, just as you would if you needed to parent a child who had a medical disability.

Chapter Tips

- Recognize your own emotions in a situation. Notice when you are frustrated or angry. Work to set aside your frustration so that you can respond from a calmer, more thoughtful frame of mind.
- Remember a word or phrase that is meaningful to you when trying to parent through your own anger or frustration.

Examples include "dignity," "this is my child," "patience," or "wisdom."
- Take a breath and maintain a body posture that shows you are ready to lead by example.
- Address the bad behavior, not your child.
- Make amends if the situation became too heated, feelings were hurt, and things were said or done that you regret.

CHAPTER 8

I Need Help

"I need help." "I can't do this by myself." "I have no idea what to do now."

It is ok to need help, and it does not mean that you are a failure or an inadequate parent to admit that you do. No one is perfect, and there is always something more to learn. The key is finding the "right" support and assistance. This likely may mean finding effective intervention in multiple areas, including medical (if needed and preferred), mental health, academic or educational, and interpersonal or social.

There is no single description of a child or person with ADHD. Even though specific criteria are used to diagnose ADHD, ADHD traits and the expression of those traits vary and are unique to each individual. You may be parenting a child who struggles daily with starting tasks, sticking with them, and finishing them with consistent quality.

You may be parenting a child who is not motivated to do anything other than his or her primary interests. Your child may have issues with emotional dysregulation such as reacting very quickly, reacting with more emotion than the situation warrants, or having difficulty shifting out of upset or angry emotions. Your child may have difficulty with regulating behavior. For example, he or she may speak or act impulsively, have a tough time stopping a preferred activity to do something else that is required, or have a hard time understanding that certain activities should be limited (eg, screen time).

Do any of these sound like your child? These specific examples are here to help you communicate with professionals about your specific needs. Stating that your child has ADHD is not enough information. For professionals to effectively help you and your child, they need to know more about your child's specific needs and the behaviors you are struggling with so they can tailor any interventions accordingly.

Another good reason for seeking professional help is that individuals with ADHD often meet diagnostic criteria for other mental health disorders. The most common are anxiety-related disorders, mood-related disorders, learning disorders, and/or other behavioral disorders. Having more than one disorder can certainly increase the need to find effective intervention for your child and family.

The situation may be further compounded if the parent has ADHD or even some ADHD traits, which is not uncommon among parents of children with ADHD. If you are in this situation, make sure that either your spouse or co-parent can provide support and help in your areas of weakness or get the additional help you need to make your parenting more effective. If you are impacted by ADHD as a parent, it is an important step to have proper supports in place for yourself.

Who Can Help?

Various types of individuals can help a child and family who are dealing with ADHD. Focusing specifically on your areas of need will help narrow your search for the type of professional and services you want.

Medical Professionals

This includes psychiatrists, primary care physicians, and nurse practitioners. These individuals are most typically the ones who make a medical assessment of the need for medication. The assessments are typically in office and often include a clinical interview and possibly completion of a checklist. Some medical professionals will request a more thorough evaluation by a psychologist if they believe diagnostic clarity is needed. Treating ADHD with medication has been extensively studied and helps in many cases. If you are considering medication, it is important to ask any and all questions you have about the medication, what to expect, and any potential side effects, both short- and long-term. You want to find a medical provider who is knowledgeable and will answer your questions so that you feel confident in the approach being taken. You'll want to understand your child's treatment and how to manage and respond to side effects should they occur.

Mental Health Professionals
This includes psychologists, counselors, social workers, and behavioral specialists who have expertise and experience working with children and adolescents with ADHD. Depending on their expertise, these individuals can focus on and address a number of different areas and needs. For example, they can assist with behavioral regulation, motivation, strategies for maintaining focus, organization, and increasing task initiation and completion. They can also offer insight about how ADHD impacts everyone in the family and the family's success, help set up behavioral programming, and offer support to decrease parent-child tension and conflict. The latter is common when children argue with a parent when asked to work on a task or activity that the child is not motivated

to complete. Working with a mental health professional can help with the communication and other skills needed to decrease these types of conflicts.

Mental health providers can also help with emotional regulation. Increasing children's understanding of their range of emotions, how their emotions impact others, and how they can manage their emotions more effectively can have a critical impact on families. Many children with ADHD do not fully understand how their emotions (especially anger) and resulting behavior affects others and why others become upset with them. In addition, children with ADHD often do not understand their full range of emotions, which often turn directly to anger, and have fewer skills to regulate such negative emotion.

An additional area of support offered by mental health professionals is assistance with understanding the subtleties of interpersonal interactions and increasing social skills. Seeing situations from another's point of view is often elusive. When this is the case, a person's actions often appear to lack empathy or compassion. An individual who sees a situation only from his or her own point of view does not understand or seem to care about another's feelings. This has a major, negative impact on interpersonal interactions and often increases frustration.

Finally, many individuals with ADHD often experience increased levels of stress and anxiety. This may be because they have an anxiety disorder in addition to ADHD, or it may be a result of their difficulties with organization, time management, and task completion. While they want and try to do well in areas that require these skills, they often struggle, which leads to negative consequences. In turn, these negative consequences create even more stress to stay organized and meet other expectations. Therefore, understanding how and why anxiety increases as well as learning strategies to manage anxiety become important. Some mental health professionals may offer cognitive-behavior therapy, an intervention that can help with anxiety, stress, and anger management.

ADHD Coaches

There is increased interest in and service availability through ADHD coaches. The typical approach of ADHD coaching is solution focused and goal oriented. ADHD coaches provide clarity with values and work consistently and persistently with individuals to provide accountability to better meet both short- and long-term goals. The beauty of ADHD coaching is that it removes the accountability component from parents—which often creates power struggles and resistance from the child—and transfers it to a neutral professional. For example, when the ADHD coach works on specific goals, such as asking about homework, the child/adolescent typically responds better than when continually asked by a parent, which the child perceives as nagging.

School Professionals
School professionals are often available to assist students who have ADHD. You may have access to a team of professionals through an informal intervention plan or through a more formal process, such as a 504 Plan (general education resources) or an IEP (special education resources). Note that specific criteria must be met to qualify for each of these types of plans, with the special education plan having a more intensive and longer qualification process. With that said, school psychologists, school social workers, school counselors, and some teachers are skilled at helping students with aspects of organization, emotional and behavioral regulation, and strategies for managing inattention. It is most helpful when the teachers and professionals who understand the most about ADHD and all know your child work together as a team. Consider asking for a meeting with your child's teacher, school counselor, principal, and other support staff if difficulties continue and there is no effective intervention or real plan in place.

Other Options
Some studies have shown that neurofeedback can be effective in treating ADHD. Neurofeedback is a non-medication approach that is a form of biofeedback. It involves gaining more control over body processes that are normally involuntary by allowing for more awareness about brain wave activity or brain states. This can increase self-awareness and skills about how to better manage these states.

Another option that is receiving more recognition is mindfulness and meditation. This approach increases awareness of mind and body in the present moment. Practicing mindfulness allows for more self-awareness and an ability to recognize emotions or reactions in a more purposeful and directed way. The result is that individuals are more consciously aware and able to respond in the present moment with more clarity or thought than they might otherwise.

"I tried, but it didn't work"
If you, your child, and your family are continuing to experience significant difficulties that are negatively impacting behavioral, emotional, interpersonal, or academic functioning, do not give up! Perseverance is called for. Not everything is a perfect fit, or at least not right away. It can take time for your

health care provider or other professional to better understand your specific needs and family dynamics. If your experience(s) was not helpful or you lacked confidence in your most recent provider, somebody else is going to be different. No health care provider is exactly the same as another. Finding the right fit may be exactly what you need to do. Persevering in finding effective professionals and resources, including targeted assistance as your child develops through different stages, can be an immeasurable assistance, and it is worth it for your child and family.

Lacking Resources

All of this sounds good, assuming you have the resources to pay for these interventions. But what if you are not in a position to pay for the ongoing assistance of a psychologist or ADHD coach? What if you have insurance, but it does not cover these services? Or what if the service provider you need does not accept insurance?

One idea is to consider setting up one, two, or three sessions with a professional with a very specific goal in mind, which may include setting up a behavior plan or motivation plan that is sustainable for your family. It may be attaining new and specific strategies that you or your child can use to assist with motivation or emotional regulation. It may be to help provide helpful book resources and additional community resources that could be ongoing.

You may also find various resources within parenting support groups. The Children and Adults with Attention Deficit/Hyperactivity Disorder (CHADD) National Resource Center on ADHD is an excellent organization with varied resources and ideas for help. Lastly, you may also consider university clinics or community mental health centers as they can offer services at a reduced rate.

You should also consider the resources already present in your life—individuals who already care and are involved with your family. These might be immediate or extended family members, friends, members of your church community or other community organizations, school personnel, or support groups. You may be able to find individuals who are able and willing to help with some respite care, tutoring, or mentoring your child. These areas of assistance can provide some relief to a stressful home situation and provide your child with another support person.

What if you have the resources, but specialized professionals are not available in your community? You may have to travel a little farther than usual to obtain services. Or, another option is virtual services or distance therapy, which is becoming more common as programs are developed. University hospital clinics, community mental health centers, ADHD coaching businesses, and some individuals in private practice are offering some distance supports. Another idea is to check with any local CHADD groups in your state or area. Individuals involved in these organizations are generally knowledgeable about local resources.

Chapter Tips

- Do not give up on professional help or assistance for your child if you have had a negative or unhelpful experience.
- Be open and consider the range of options and supports available to you.
- Be clear about what you are looking for and your specific needs.
- Continue to communicate with your professional providers, school personnel, and others involved with your child.
- Continue to seek resources if you are feeling overwhelmed or if things are not improving.

CHAPTER 9

I'm an Over-Functioning Parent

A poignant consideration for all parents, but especially for those raising a child with ADHD is "how much am I helping and how much am I enabling?" Many parents do more for their child with ADHD than for their other children and they do more than they think they should given their child's age and other abilities. However, parents feel stuck in a cycle because without their help or intervention, day-to-day activities are either not finished on time or not finished at all. Common activities include getting ready for school, getting to school on time, finishing tasks or homework, and keeping things even semi-organized so important items can be found again.

Individuals with ADHD lag developmentally in the ability to self-regulate, usually in more than one area. These include cognitive (eg, organization, focus and attention, working memory, prioritization), behavioral (eg, impulsivity, lack of inhibition), and emotional regulation (eg, emotional inhibition, emotional self-control, anger management). Because of how these difficulties show up in everyday situations, many parents feel compelled to "pick up the slack." If you didn't, things would simply not get done on time and then there would be a bigger problem to solve, or you would be stuck in repeating cycles of emotional meltdown and conflict. However, on the other hand, if you establish a pattern of essentially taking over your child's responsibilities, is that really helping? What are the long-term consequences? Will your child be dependent on someone forever?

When children with ADHD do not follow through or take needed responsibility, a commonly heard comment is, "just let them fail, they will learn." While this perspective and advice *can* be true, it doesn't always completely work for a child with ADHD. You can allow your child to "fail" by not helping with organization or homework completion, but your child is likely to do something similar next term. You can let your child be responsible for his or her own things, but inevitably something will get lost or forgotten. You either have to become involved, or the child will go without.

I'm an Over-Functioning Parent

Failure is not always the wisest teacher in ADHD. The fact is that your child probably knows exactly what he or she needs to do but lacks the executive functioning abilities to do so. Or your child may have failed and doesn't seem to learn how to be more organized, attentive, or self-regulated. So, what other choices do you have?

I am glad you asked.

Parenting Persona

Returning to your overall values and goals is a very important place to begin. Think about your overall goals for your child and hold on to them. Now this time, consider how to incorporate those values into your parenting choices. What do you value, and what do you want when considering your relationship with your child? Do you want to be the task master, the disciplinarian, the cool parent? You likely do all of these in some capacity, but consider what type of parent you want to be overall. In a fuller sense, do you want to be the enabler ("I'll do that for you"), the excuse maker ("you know she has ADHD"), the parent who over functions ("I'll do that and that and that"), or the parent who nags ("seriously, aren't you done yet?")? All of these personas and parenting habits have positive and negative aspects.

When most people really think about the type of parent they would like to be, they want to be a parent who is both understanding and insightful. A parent who understands the developmental lags that the child is experiencing, but who is also wise to manipulation and enabling. You may also want to be the parent who has effective strategies and wise responses to day-to-day challenges and overarching struggles. And parents universally want to have a healthy and loving relationship with their children who they can watch grow and become more independent and capable. You want to be the parent who gives your children the best childhood you can and provide a solid foundation so that they may thrive and prosper in their adult life.

If this is you, an important concept to consider and practice is scaffolding.

Scaffolding

Scaffolding is a very popular educational concept and practice. Scaffolding is providing just enough support for students to help them move from where they are to the next step in their learning. In teaching, there is a "sweet spot" where students have some knowledge, but then with just the right combination of factors present, they experience real learning—an "aha" moment—when they move a step forward in their understanding or skill level.

I'm an Over-Functioning Parent

In education, teachers use different strategies such as modeling, coaching, providing relevant examples, giving partial answers or cues, or working together to come up with a solution.

In parenting, we also scaffold. We work to help our children learn important concepts and ways to live and behave. We provide scaffolding to assist in everyday experiences to teach our children to understand what works and what doesn't. We try to teach them step by step when learning any new skill or gaining a new concept.

The assumption with scaffolding is that as you model, teach, and work together with children, they continue to learn. However, it doesn't quite work that way with a child with ADHD. So, you also have to consider what else *you* need to learn. Consider yourself as needing scaffolding. You have been trying something one way, and it has not been working. So, you need to consider what other supports or strategies might improve or move the situation in a positive direction. It is also important to recognize that when a child has ADHD, a particular support or strategy may work beautifully one day but not the next. Don't despair! This is typical, and just lets you know that you need more than one tool in your toolkit.

Scenario

Mia is a bright 8th-grade student who has difficulties with time management. She has a hard time getting started and then takes anywhere from 10 to 30 minutes to engage enough to get any work completed. Her parents have been task masters, staying on her from start to finish to get it done. When they do not, Mia typically works throughout the night trying to finish her homework and may forget some of what she needs to do. Mia's teachers have recommended that her parents allow her to be more independent, but when they do, the result is much more stress for everyone, especially for Mia.

After years of doing this the same way they always have, Mia's parents decided to try a more balanced approach. With the help of a professional, they had important discussions with Mia to identify her feelings and thoughts about how her work is completed—her struggles, her goals, her intentions, and her commitments. From this, they started a system in which Mia was responsible to get organized and start her homework, follow through, and turn it in on time. However, they also determined where they needed to support Mia within this system, such as by helping with motivation to get started, asking for some accountability throughout the process, and coaching for organization and follow through. While Mia's parents are now supporting her in ways that are needed, they are sharing responsibility with her in hopes that her future adult self will be able to manage on her own, or at least know what supports she needs to manage on her own.

Flexibility

Another important aspect in finding the right parenting balance is flexibility. Flexibility involves not only considering changing how you do something as a parent, but also how you think about it. Be open to other ways of approaching a situation or problem. For example, can you think of a new way to approach a child who resists eating breakfast or who resists using a pencil for math? Be flexible in how you think about all aspects of this issue. What are you currently doing that has not worked time and time again? Is there another way to say it? Is there another solution? Is it something that can be let go? Don't get stuck in the "my child just won't listen or do what I say" mindset. There is always another way. Stay flexible in your thinking and be willing to try it another way.

Another point to remember is that inflexibility is a common trait in individuals with ADHD. Most often, individuals with ADHD think of doing something in only one way and are challenged by coming up with multiple ways to solve a problem. So, if you strive to be flexible in your approach, not only are you likely to solve a problem or at least improve a situation, but you are also modeling flexibility for your child. And in doing so, you are teaching (or at least exposing) your child how to be more flexible in approaching situations or problems. Your child may resist initially, but your continued efforts will help your child in the long run. Think about how invaluable having some flexibility skills will be to your child as an adult.

Here are a few areas that might call for some flexibility:

- How you think about a problem or issue: "My child just won't listen to me" versus maybe what I am saying does not resonate with him or her.
- How you present yourself in a situation and consequently how it is interpreted by your child
- What behavior is being reinforced: What behavior does your child show that actually gets a desired result? For example, does your child get a positive reaction from you

when she completes her homework the way you tell her to do it? Or, does she get a positive reaction from you when she has engaged in her own problem solving?

Scenario

Samantha is constantly thinking about how to get her son, Gerald, ready on time in the morning, including having eaten his breakfast before it's time to leave for school. Some mornings go well, but others do not. She is constantly reminding him how much time he has, how much time is left, and what he still needs to do. This annoys Gerald, and he talks back when Samantha reminds and prods him. This scenario repeats over and over... What else can Samantha do?

Samantha decides to try another method to assist with time management. She did a search on Google and found that some parents use a time timer, some use apps as an accountability tool for the morning routine, and some have tried using a behavior reinforcement system for having all steps finished at a certain time. She is not sure what will work best for Gerald, but she is willing to be flexible and think outside her normal box, which has only led to frustration for everyone.

Am I Done Yet?

No. I cannot say it any simpler than that. You are not done. But you love your child and you are your child's best support and advocate. The goal is to parent in developmentally appropriate ways for *your* child. Given your child's age, he or she may need typical parenting in some areas but not others. You may have to parent in a unique way considering your child's specific range of abilities. As your child grows, you can work into offering advice or support when they ask for it and need it. When your child is a young adult, you hope to be in a supportive role on the sideline, because they will be living their own life and making decisions as they see fit. The hope is that you have done enough scaffolding, honest supporting, and working with your child over the years that, in their maturity, they realize and have learned how to manage their own challenges with ADHD.

Chapter Tips

- Recognize when you are doing too much for you child and consider how to share the responsibility in a way that matches your child's current abilities.

I'm an Over-Functioning Parent

- Recognize if your child has learned that you will take on the task, and begin shifting the responsibility back to your child, even if initially it takes more effort and time.
- Consider how you can "scaffold" or teach by provide modeling, reminders, or cooperative efforts.
- Remain flexible in your thinking. If something has not worked or worked well, consider how you can change it or try it another way.
- Day-to-day parenting is your ultimate teacher.

CHAPTER 10

My Child Is a Gift

Let's be honest. Some days, you may not think that your child is a gift, particularly when in the middle of something challenging, annoying, or downright disappointing. But even in those moments, deep down you love your child and want to do the best you can for him or her.

What You Convey

Stop to consider what you think about your child. What are your opinions, attitudes, and thoughts about your child as a whole person? It's true that sometimes your thoughts may be less than positive or hopeful. But keep in mind that whatever you actually think about a person is what you ultimately communicate, either directly or indirectly. Consider what you most frequently think your child is to you. What traits or characteristics come to mind? How do you describe your child? What do other family members know that you think about your child? These are clues to what you cultivate in your actions and what, ultimately, your actions are showing.

So, stop and think about what you really think about your child and what you think most frequently. Anyone can get caught up in negative thought processes: "My child is my payback considering how I acted as a child" or "I just want to get this kid through high school" or "My child is the most stubborn person." However, be honest and acknowledge what comes to mind when you consider what your child really is to you.

Now, think "_____ *(insert your child's name)* is a gift." _____ is a gift whom I have been given. How do you respond to this gift? How do you interact with this gift? Do you show gratitude for what this child brings to your life? Challenges, sure, but also joy and the connection that comes from loving a child and being loved in return. If you think about your child in this way, it can change your mindset and how you approach dealing with aspects of your child's personality. It can also change deep feelings of frustration or possibly resentment that you may have. When you think about a person or a situation as a gift, you also open your mind to the ways in which you yourself can grow, change, and learn. Children have a unique way of challenging your personal traits and weaknesses. Your child is a gift in different forms, not only to bring love and connection, but also to help you grow as a person and a parent.

When you say to your child, "I see you as a great gift" or maybe "you are the greatest gift to me," watch what happens. How would you feel if someone said that to you? Let that soak in. This one statement, spoken genuinely and sincerely, can have a very deep effect. Wow.

I Don't Feel It

If your relationship with your child has some deep or challenging aspects, maybe you are not in a place to consider a more positive outcome in the moment. Maybe it doesn't seem natural. But maybe you are in a place to begin to think about a shift in thinking. How do you really want to think about your child? Is there something better than a gift? If you do not feel as strong of an emotional connection with your child as you would like to because of difficulties with ADHD or other behavioral issues, then begin by focusing on aspects of your child that you *are* grateful for. Focus on the positives about your child. As a beginning, note and be sure to remember any progress and positive growth that your child has made.

You Are the Teacher

Remember that you are your child's ultimate teacher. Your child learns from you every day and will remember how you respond and what you model. But don't be nervous about that. No one is a perfect parent. We can always repair a situation when needed. However, keep in mind that your overall responses and what you show and give of yourself will be remembered and often modeled. If you remember that you are setting the example, it will help you to be thoughtful about your actions and intentions. Even when children become adolescents and seek their friends, they still watch how their parents handle situations as a guide, especially when there is a strong connection.

Being the best teacher that you can be for managing day-to-day life this is more important than any grade or performance.

You Can Do This!

It's time I get to be your cheerleader! We all need encouragement, reminders, and focus points to stay positive and keep up the hard work. So here goes...

You can do this because your child is depending on you. You have your child's best interests at heart, more than anyone else. You have more experience and insight into your child than anyone else in the world, including your child. Even though your child may not believe that or understand it, you know it's true.

You can do this because you know your child is worth it. All the struggles, all the effort, all the energy are well worth it when you consider that you are raising a human being who will eventually go off and live a life outside your care—an independent life that will influence others, someone who may have children of their own someday. What you provide as a parent cannot be bought or taken away from your child, so make it the best you have to offer.

You can do this because you intimately know all your child's capabilities. Think about what you truly like and appreciate about your child and know that these qualities or characteristics are likely present and even magnified in your child because of you. Strive to nurture these strengths in your child.

You can do this because you love your child. Your child is a gift and has been entrusted in your care. In the deepest sense, you want your child's life and their life experience to be fulfilling and rich.

You know in your heart that being a genuine, loving, and deeply giving parent will result in rich returns from your children. Although you may not experience immediate benefits from your efforts and sacrifices today, be assured that your children and your children's children, as well as others they encounter in their lives, will be much richer for your years of support and guidance. Parenting is part of the circle of life and is best done out of love. Keep it up!

Chapter Tips

- Think "my child is a gift." Let that sink in and see how it feels.
- Consider this when frustrated with your child to help lead you to wise reactions and decisions.
- Shed negative thinking about your child that doesn't fit your values.
- Know that wise and loving parenting has overall and overarching benefits.
- Remember that you are a gift to your child!